# NP
# Notebook

*nurse*

{ners} n.  a scrub wearing, smile bringing, life saving rockstar who lives to heal and loves to encourage.

*See also*: SUPERHERO

This book belongs to:

_____

DATE: _____

DATE: _____

DATE: _____

DATE: _____

DATE: _____

DATE: _____

DATE: _____

DATE: _____

DATE: _____

DATE: _____

DATE: _____

DATE: _____

DATE: _____

DATE: _____

DATE: _____

DATE: _____

DATE: _____

DATE: _____

DATE: _____

DATE: _____

DATE: _____

DATE: _____

DATE: _____

DATE: _____

DATE: _____

DATE: _____

DATE: _____

DATE: _____

DATE: _____

DATE: _____

DATE: _____

DATE: _____

DATE: _____

DATE: _____

DATE: _____

DATE: _____

DATE: _____

DATE: _____

DATE: _____

DATE: _____

DATE: _____

DATE: _____

DATE: _____

DATE: _____

DATE: _____

DATE: _____

DATE: _____

DATE: _____

DATE: _____

# Quotes from Patients

Date

Who?

Where?

Quote

# Quotes from Patients

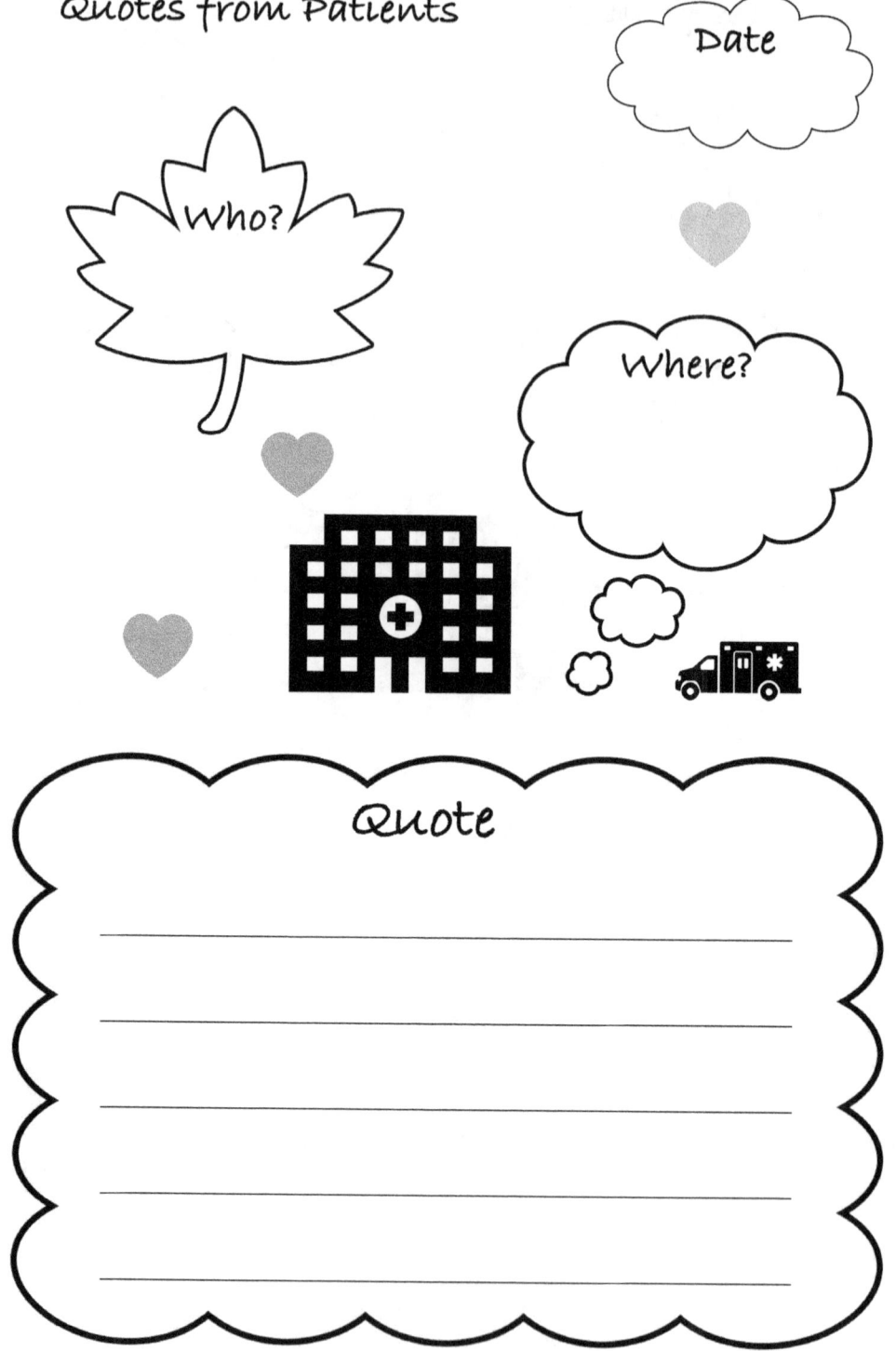

Date

Who?

Where?

Quote

_____
_____
_____
_____

Quotes from Patients

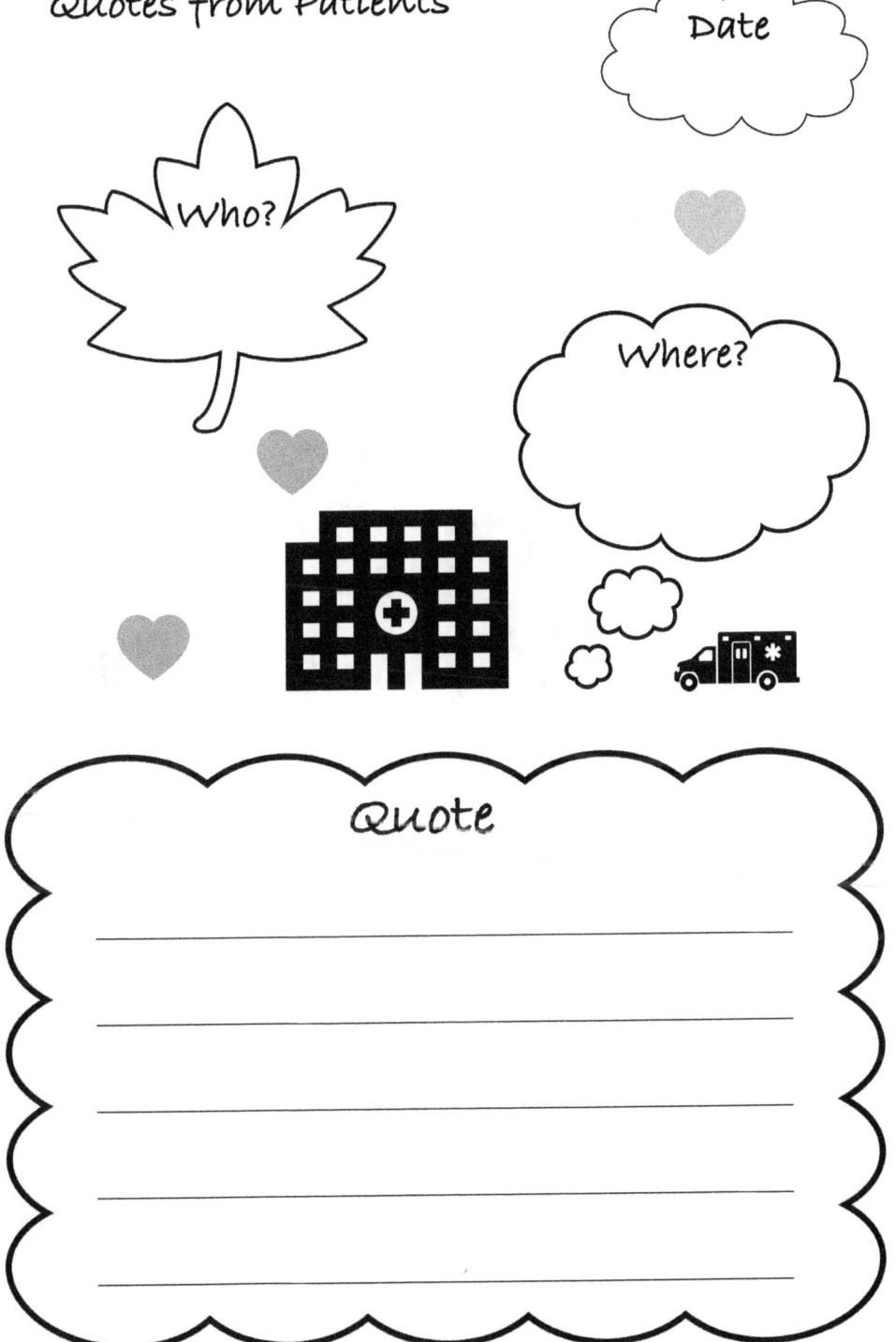

Date

Who?

Where?

Quote

# Quotes from Patients

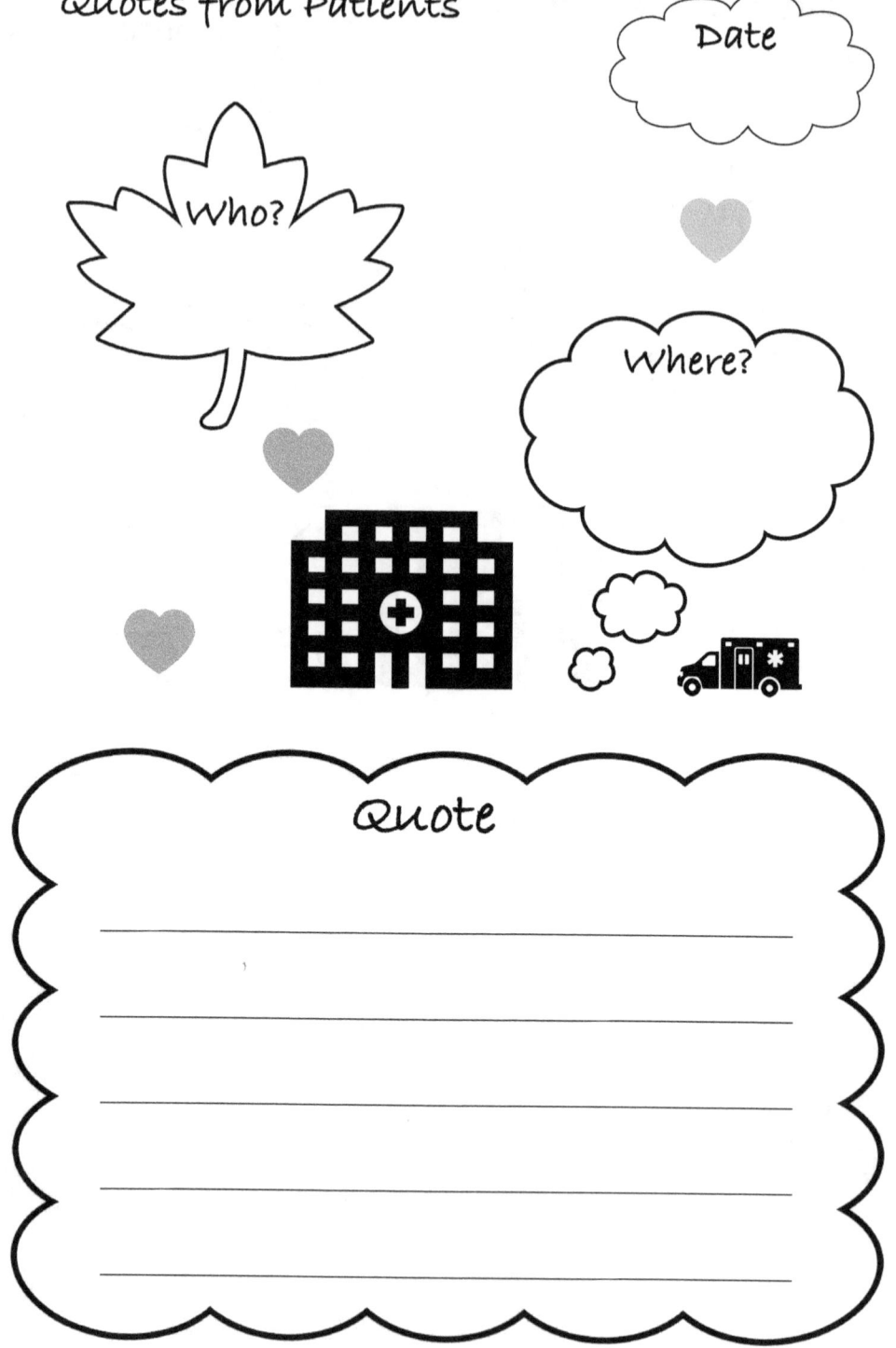

Date

Who?

Where?

Quote

# Coloring Section

I Had Fun Once,Then
I Went To Nursing School

# Ativan A Nurse's Best Friend

# Eat.
# Sleep.
# Nurse.
# Repeat

# DO NOT MAKE ME SEDATE YOU.

# Best Nurse Ever

I'VE SEEN MORE
PRIVATES
THAN THE ARMY
GENERAL

# Nurse Squad

# If You're Happy and You Know It, It's Your Meds